HEALTH FOR THE PACIFIC 6

Safety

in Papua New Guinea

by Richard Jones

OXFORD
UNIVERSITY PRESS
AUSTRALIA & NEW ZEALAND

Contents

Foreword

The lack of clear, simple and accurate information about good health contributes to poor health in any society.

This series is intended to educate by highlighting important health and safety issues that are affecting the lives of young men, women and children in the Pacific region.

Risk-taking behaviour, natural disasters, emergency situations and safety issues contribute to ill health. Therefore, there is a need to educate our people about how to keep safe. Young people need to know the risks to which they are exposed and the preventive measures that can be taken. Life skills play an important part in avoiding risk and dealing with unsafe or emergency situations.

Health and safety is everyone's concern.

Acknowledgments

There are many risks to the safety of young men and women: natural disasters, violence, unsafe transport, risky behaviour and dangers in the environment and community. Young people need to learn how to minimise these risks and how to deal with unsafe situations in the home, school, community and wider environment. Drowning, road accidents, burns, violence and sexual abuse are all very real risks, and learning life skills can protect young people from them.

This text is written to support the teaching of Personal Development in Papua New Guinea primary schools from Grade 6 onwards. It is a booklet for students and a resource book for teachers.

I would like to thank the many dedicated teachers and teacher trainers in the Department of Education who teach life skills to their students, and who help guide young people through the challenges in their life. I dedicate this book to them.

Richard Jones

Notes for teachers

This booklet has been written for Upper Primary and Lower Secondary school students studying the Personal Development subject. The knowledge, skills and attitudes developed in the text contribute to these learning outcomes from Personal Development:

Personal Development Grades 6–8

6.2.4 Identify rules and demonstrate safety procedures in play and games

6.4.8 Identify potentially hazardous situations at school, home and the community

6.5.2 Describe the process of making decisions

7.2.4 Develop procedures for dealing with unsafe or emergency situations

7.4.7 Propose ways of responding to situations that threaten personal health and safety

7.4.8 Describe behaviours that affect personal and community safety

7.5.2 Outline the positive and negative results of making choices

8.2.4 Demonstrate behaviours that influence personal safety and the safety of others in games and play

8.4.6 Outline health issues that are of concern to young people

8.4.8 Develop strategies to respond to unsafe or risky situations

There are also strong curriculum links with Community Living and Health in Lower Primary, and Social Science and Making a Living in the Upper Primary syllabus.

There are many activities in the text for the students to complete and discuss. These can be used for self-study, or as teaching and learning activities in class. They are designed for maximum student participation and the development of life skills.

Introduction

There are many challenges for young men and women growing up in our country. Personal and community safety are two of these challenges that have an important impact on our health.

Many young people are put at risk by situations in their community. These can be dangers in the home, the school and the environment. There can be natural dangers such as flooded rivers and snakebite, or human risks such as bullying and road accidents. Young people may also have to deal with emergency situations such as natural disasters.

Risks to safety can be physical, mental or emotional. However, all young people and their families and friends can work to reduce these risks. They can do this by learning key life skills, and important information about how to deal quickly and sensibly with safety issues and unsafe situations.

Young people need to know the facts about unsafe and emergency situations. They need to know how to make safe and careful decisions to protect their health and the health of others. Risky behaviour can put them at risk of injury, harm or even death. Many families and children have been hurt through a lack of life skills and basic knowledge about safety.

The knowledge and life skills you will learn from this book can help you keep yourself healthy and safe, and improve the health of your community.

Chapter 1 What is safety?

When someone is safe, they are not at risk from their environment or from people. Staying safe is important for your health and happiness and for having a long and productive life.

Many of the situations young people face in their lives are unsafe. They are at risk of harm. These unsafe situations and hazards are common in our community. They can happen in the home, in the garden, at school, on the road, at sea and in the bush.

Sometimes young people and their families face emergency situations. These are not as common as unsafe situations, but can lead to injury or even death. Papua New Guinea is at risk of many natural disasters because of its location. The country is vulnerable to floods, earthquakes, cyclones, tsunamis, volcanic eruptions and bushfires.

Families can also face emergency situations in the community, such as house fires, violence and serious illness. It is important that we are all prepared for these situations and know how to deal with them quickly and safely.

Activity 1·1

Work with a partner to brainstorm the unsafe and emergency situations people might face in their communities. For example:

Unsafe situations – drunken youths, wild animals, road accidents

Emergency situations – floods, fire, landslides

Life skills

Life skills protect us from harm in many ways. In unsafe and emergency situations, you might have to make quick decisions to protect your life and the lives of others. For example, if you are on the beach and you see the sea water quickly running away, you should know that a tsunami is coming. You have to run away to higher ground and warn others.

There are also unsafe situations that could lead to harm. Life skills such as decision-making, critical thinking, first-aid skills and assertiveness help to protect you and others from harm. Knowing what to do in the event of an emergency and having a plan of action can help you through an unsafe situation.

It is also important to be able to recognise situations and individuals that might put you at risk of physical or sexual assault. You might meet people who are violent or drunk. Some people would like to touch or hurt you. There are people who might want to have sex with you, even if you do not want sex. These are all unsafe situations and you have to know how to protect yourself. Life skills such as assertiveness and good decision-making will help you. For example, if an uncle tried to touch you sexually or made you feel uncomfortable or scared, you should know that you need to tell a trusted adult or police officer. You should know how to say "no" in a strong and assertive way. You might even need some self-defence skills.

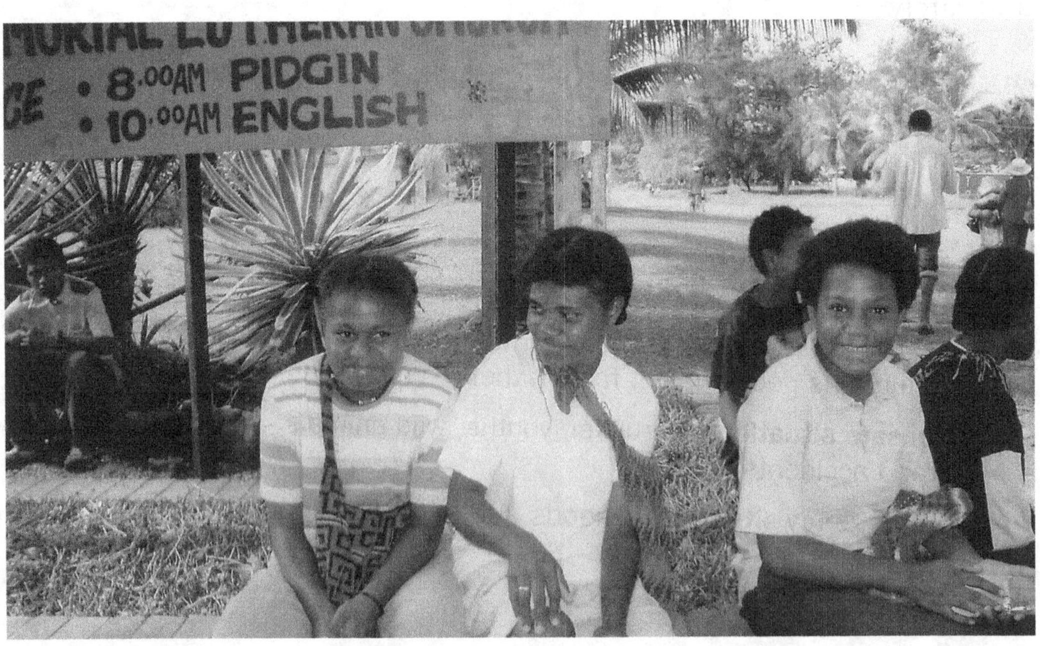

Unsafe situations

These are situations that could possibly lead to harm:

- road traffic and crossing a road
- boat travel
- crossing a river
- cooking on an open fire
- using knives or axes
- playing rough games or playing in the bush
- collecting water from a well
- being alone with someone you don't know or a family member who makes you feel uncomfortable or scared
- using fertilisers, poisons and pesticides
- using electrical equipment
- medicines that aren't used properly or stored safely
- bullying
- visiting places where people drink or gamble.

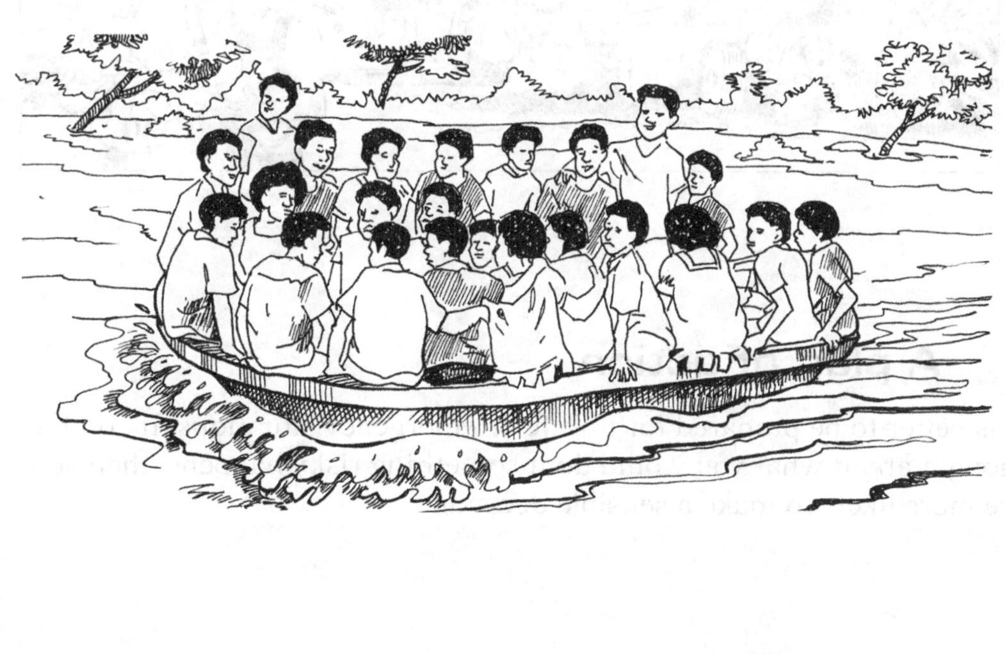

Emergency situations

These are situations that are very dangerous:

- road accidents
- boat accidents
- injuries, burns or poisoning
- natural disasters (volcanoes, earthquakes, tsunamis, floods, cyclones, bushfires)
- drunken people
- people who want to have sex with you or touch you without your permission
- violent people or tribal fights
- wild animals like snakes, stonefish or wild pigs
- serious sudden illnesses like malaria, heart attacks, asthma attacks or constant diarrhoea.

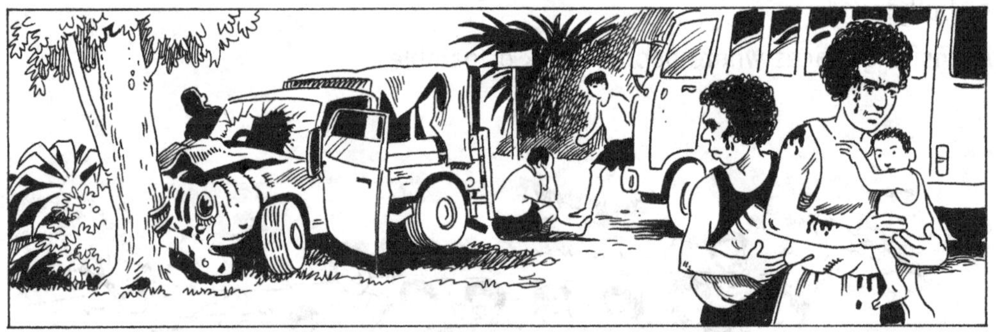

A plan of action

It is better to be prepared for unsafe or emergency situations. If you have thought about what you would do if something risky happens, then you are more likely to make a sensible decision.

What if?

- You walk into the house and see your little sister has eaten some of the malaria medicine, thinking it was sweets...
- You walk down to school and find the river is flooding and full of muddy water. It is blocking your normal path to school...
- A boy in your class threatens you when the teacher is out of the room, and makes you give him your pen...
- There is a fight between two drunken men in the village...
- You are playing in the forest. You fall over and cut your hand. It is bleeding badly...
- You are in the classroom and there is a powerful earthquake. Everyone is frozen in fear...

Activity 1·2

What would you do in these situations? Discuss your answers with a friend to see if they have the same responses. Then work with your friend to write about two more emergency situations.

1. What is the risk in each scenario?
2. What is the best decision to make in each scenario? Why?
3. What are the alternative choices?
4. What might happen if you made a different choice?

Chapter 2 Staying safe with people

The biggest risk to young men and women is always other people. Most people we meet in our lives are friendly and caring, but there are some people who might want to do us harm. Your safety depends on spotting these risks and knowing what to do in that situation. Your life may depend on it.

People you can trust

It is important that you know who can help you if you feel unsafe or if there is an emergency. This person has to be trustworthy and someone you know well and who knows you well. This person has to be a good role model and someone who would be able to make good decisions.

> Remember, you have the right to safety and health. No one is allowed to hurt you in any way. There will be many people who will help you if you need them. There are also non-governmental organisations that can help young people who need support. A list of these organisations and their contact details can be found at the back of this book.

Who would you turn to first in an emergency or unsafe situation?

- a sensible friend
- your parents
- a trusted older brother or sister
- a trusted uncle or aunt
- a grandparent
- your teacher or head teacher
- your local police officer
- a local health worker
- your school-based counsellor
- your pastor or chaplain.

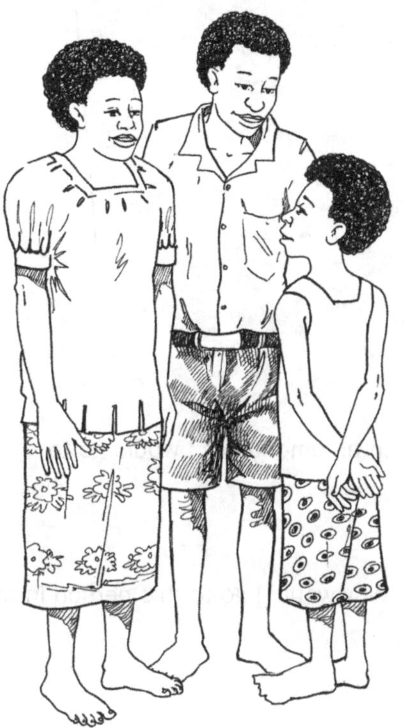

Activity 2·1

1. Who would you go to in an emergency or if you thought your safety was threatened? Why?
2. Use the template on the next page to write a personal profile of this person. Don't forget to tell this person that you would go to them in an emergency.
3. Who else could you go to if this person was not available? Make a list.

PERSONAL PROFILE

In an emergency I would go to:

Why would I go to this person in an emergency?

What personal qualities does this person have?

Where is this person located?

If this person has a phone number, write it here:

Risky times and places

It is possible to avoid trouble by avoiding risky places and times in your community. These might be places where people are often drunk or places that are dark and quiet. There might be times when there are lots of people gathering together, such as dances or market days. Often there are problems in communities on paydays. Other risky places could be roads and rivers. For example, sea travel is risky late at night or if the boat operator is drunk.

Remember, most people are good and caring. If you feel unsafe or threatened by people, you must get away from the situation and tell someone you trust. This person will help you.

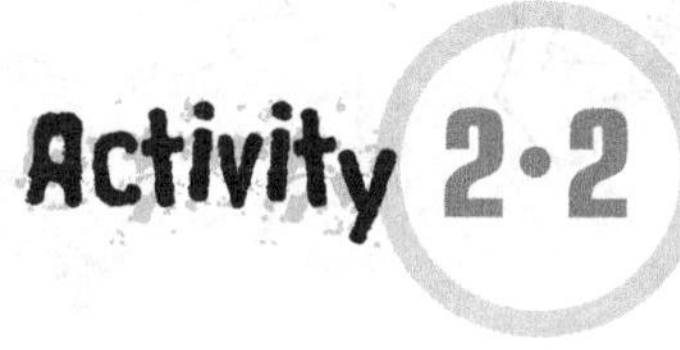

Activity 2·2

1 Draw a sketch map of your community and label the places where you might be at risk from people. Also write which times are risky. For example, the market is safe in the morning but there is a risk of being robbed late in the afternoon.

2 Now compare your map with a friend's. Are there some places and times that are riskier for boys or girls? Why?

Risks from other people for boys and young men

"I was walking back from school alone and a group of older boys were waiting along the bush track. They were smoking spak brus and I was afraid. They shouted over to me."

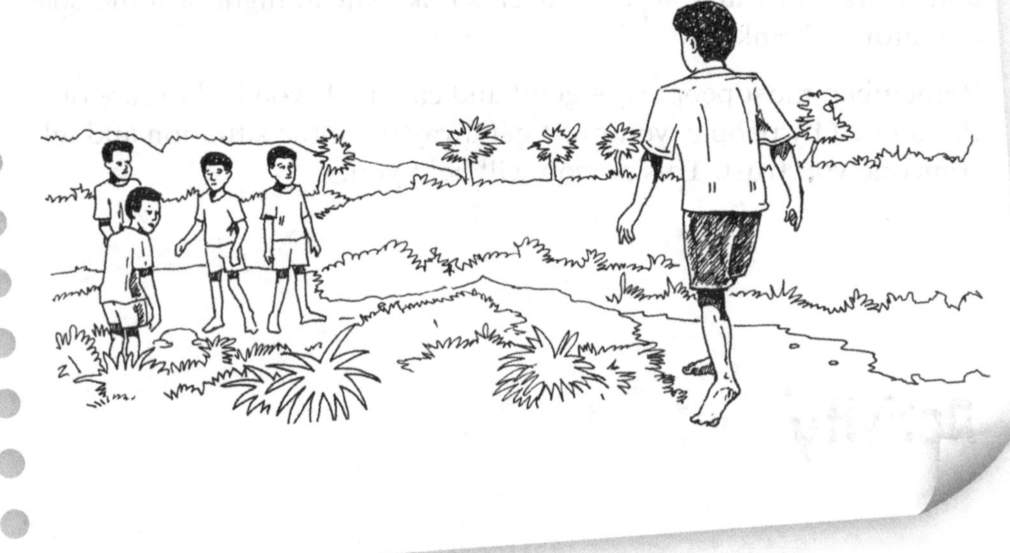

There are many risks from people to young men and boys. Violence and robbery are both dangerous situations. Boys can also be the victims of bullying and threats or rape and sexual assault. Young men can be caught up in tribal fights and payback. They might feel that they have a traditional obligation to take part, even though it is against the law. Tribal fights damage the development of the community and the country.

Young men are also under peer pressure to smoke, use marijuana and drink home-brew or beer. Young men sometimes feel they have to be strong, aggressive and sexually active to be respected. This is not true: it is dangerous peer pressure. Having sex too young, fighting or getting drunk puts you at risk of harm.

It is important that young men, their families and their communities work together to make growing up safe and healthy for young men.

Risks from other people for girls and young women

"I had a wantok staying in my house. He would always look at me in a strange and scary way. I was nervous about being alone in the house with him. Then one day he had been drinking and he tried to force me to have sex with him. He touched my body and made me cry. I told my father and he threw the uncle out of the house."

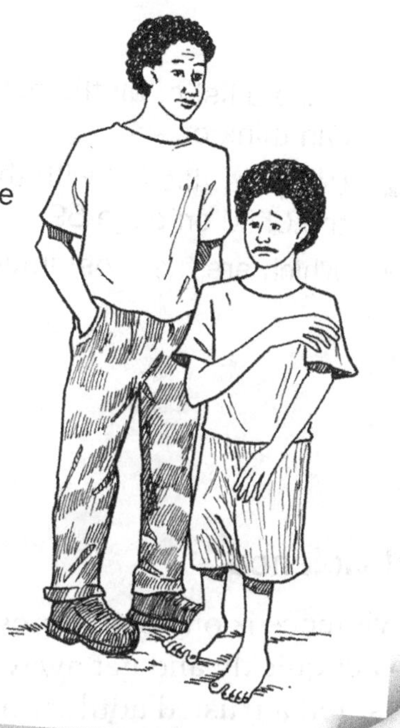

Sadly, girls and young women are vulnerable to violence, robbery, rape and sexual assault. Some men in PNG do not respect women. Some men touch women or girls in a way that scares them. They might touch their bottom, breasts, legs or sexual organs or speak to them in a sexual way. This is sexual assault and harassment. It is a crime.

Young women are also vulnerable to peer pressure to drink alcohol, use drugs and have sex too young. Young women and girls are especially vulnerable to dropping out of school and being used as slaves around the house (cooking, cleaning, working in the garden, etc.) rather than getting an education. They are also at risk of marrying too young, having sex for money, or unplanned pregnancy.

It is vital for the future of our country that girls are respected, educated and cared for by the community and their family. The community should work to keep all children and young people safe from harm from others. All young people need to learn how to identify people, places and times that are risky to their safety and learn skills for keeping safe.

Activity 2·3

1 Make a list of all the rights of children and young people that you can think of.
2 Compare this list with the Universal Declaration on the Rights of the Child on page 59.
3 Which are the most important rights for children in PNG? Why?

Sexual violence

Sexual violence is one of the most dangerous situations you can face. You need to act quickly and get away from the situation as soon as possible. You must tell a trusted adult straight away. It is sometimes difficult to tell someone but it is important to do this.

If you cannot run away, the best strategy is to make as much noise as possible and try and hurt your attacker. Kicking or punching them between the legs, stabbing your fingers into their eyes or throat, pushing them away, biting them, kicking their kneecaps and screaming loudly may work. This is called self-defence. Your local police officer or a martial arts club can teach you these skills.

Violent conflict

Violence is common in some of our communities. It can happen during a robbery, or because someone is drunk and aggressive. Violence can also be caused by jealousy or traditional payback and tribal fights. The best strategy is to get away from the situation as quickly as possible until everything calms down. Call for help and back away from the violent person.

If you cannot get away, or you want to try and calm the person down, speak calmly and softly. Show your hands and keep a safe distance away. Keep yourself safe. Make eye contact with the person. If the person attacks you, use your self-defence skills and then try to get away.

Robbery

Being robbed is very scary and you will need to make a quick decision. If the robber is armed with a gun or a knife and you cannot run away, it is better to give up your bilum or money. Try to make a lot of noise and yell for help. You should also be prepared to use your self-defence skills.

Resisting peer pressure

Peer pressure can put you at risk. You must be assertive and confident to resist peer pressure. Just because your friends are drinking alcohol or having unsafe sex, this does not mean you have to put yourself at risk too. Your behaviour and choices might have serious consequences. For example, sex without a condom could lead to HIV/AIDS, STIs or unplanned pregnancy.

There are many strategic life skills for resisting peer pressure:

- Say "no" and give a strong reason.
- Make an excuse and leave the unsafe situation.
- Use assertive body language and eye contact.
- Be prepared to be independent and different.
- Feel good about your decision-making and values.

The tribal fight

You are a young man. The men of your village are getting ready to attack the people in the next community. Your friends at school are all running to join in. What would you do? Why? What might the consequences be?

The market man

You are a young woman in a crowded market and you feel a man pressing close to you. He is touching you in a scary way. Maybe he is trying to rob you. Maybe it is something worse. What would you do? Why? What might the consequences be?

Boasting

You are a male grade 8 student. Your best friend is boasting of having sex with a girl at the school. He is telling you all about it. Then he says he knows a girl who wants to have sex with you. What would you do? Why? What might the consequences be?

Sorcery

You are walking home from the market when you see a fight. A man is beating a woman badly and accusing her of casting a spell on him. You know both of them. She runs towards you and hides behind you. What would you do? Why? What might the consequences be?

Drunken dad

Your father returns home on payday and he is drunk and aggressive. Your mother and brothers and sisters are all scared. He throws a plate of food across the room. What would you do? Why? What might the consequences be?

Activity 2·4

- Read the case studies on the opposite page with a partner.
- Work out what you would do in each situation and what the consequences might be.

Safety tips:

- Don't travel alone – always move around in a group.
- Don't walk around late at night.
- Tell people where you are going and what time you expect to be back.
- Give trusted people your phone number and get the phone numbers of people who could help you in an emergency.
- Don't carry too much money or show your mobile phone.
- Carry a whistle to use if you are attacked.

Chapter 3 Safety at play

Everyone loves to play. Keeping safe when you are playing is important. Many formal games and sports have rules to make sure players don't get hurt. Even with these rules, sometimes accidents and injuries occur, so you need to know what to do if someone gets hurt during play.

The *Basic First Aid* book in this series has more skills you can learn. You can also learn more from a health worker, teacher or a non-governmental organisation like the Red Cross.

Keeping safe in sport

First aid kit

Most village teams have a simple first aid kit. Your school should also have one. It will need a bandage, ice pack, latex gloves, plasters, iodine, scissors, tweezers and clean water.

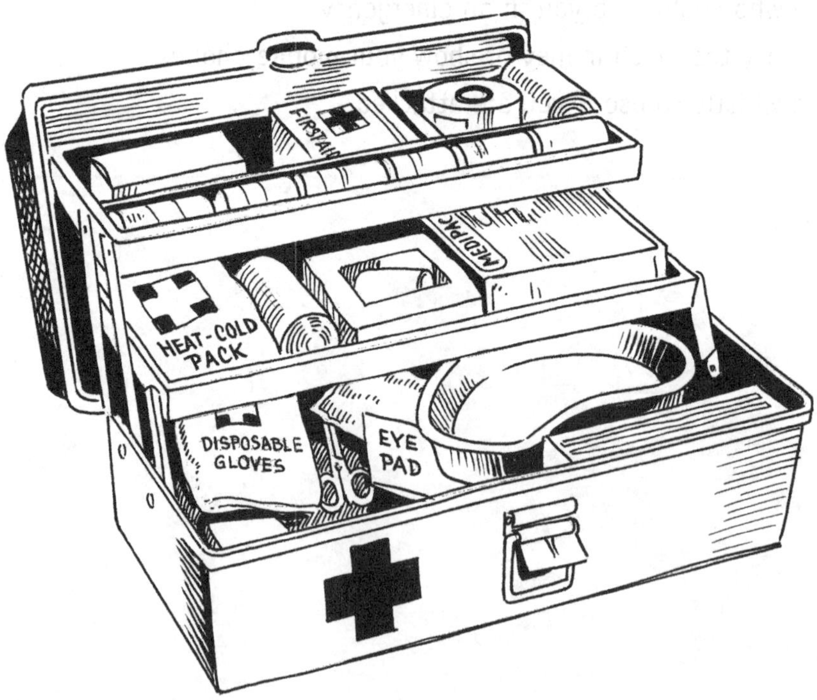

Check the pitch

Always walk around the pitch or field to make sure there are no bottles, cans, broken glass, sticks, sharp stones or animal faeces lying about. Fill in any holes or animal burrows, and make sure the posts and nets are secure.

Protective clothing

Rugby players and boxers need mouthguards to protect their teeth. Soccer players need shin pads too. Some sports need studded boots so make sure the studs are not too sharp or worn dangerously. If some players do not have studs or shoes, then everyone should play in bare feet.

Stretching and warming up

Before the game, all the players should warm up by stretching and jogging. This gets their muscles, heart and joints ready for exercise. Hold the stretches for about ten to fifteen seconds and don't bounce up and down when stretching.

Play by the rules

Most injuries are accidental but sometimes players deliberately hurt each other. You will be sent off if you cheat or hurt another player. Play by the rules of the game, respect and listen to the referee, and keep yourself under control all the time. If you lose your temper, you will lose the game!

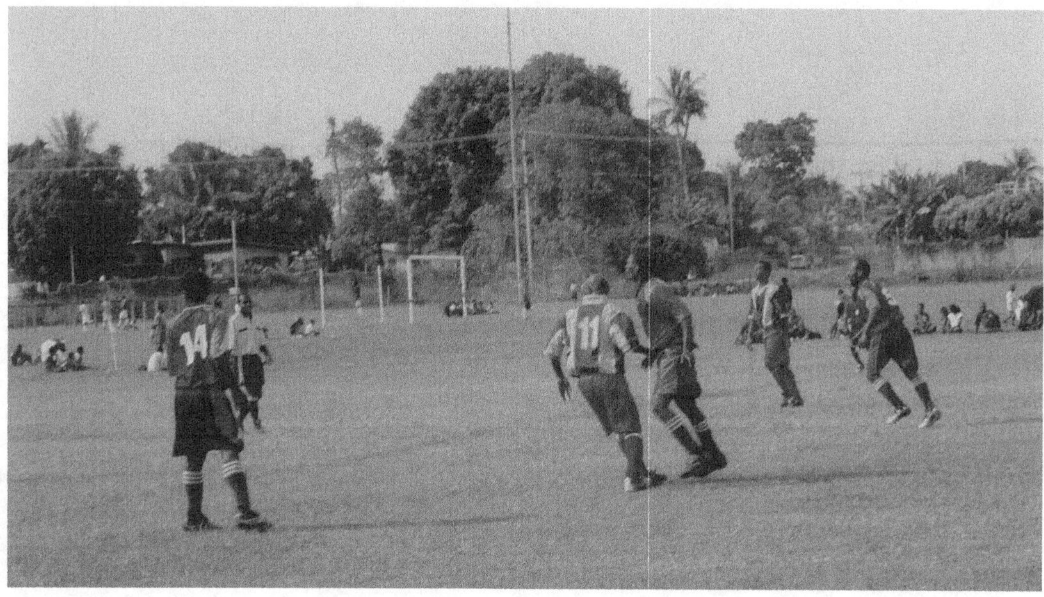

Stop for injuries

Stop playing if someone is injured. The game should stop while the injury is sorted out. No one should play if they are injured or bleeding. It is safe to clean up someone else's blood if you don't have any open wounds on your own hands. You will not be infected with HIV. If you have latex gloves, then you should use them.

Bleeding wounds should be stopped with firm pressure and bandaged. Head wounds bleed a lot. If the person feels dizzy or faint, lie them down. Try to raise the bleeding limb above the height of the head. Some wounds might need stitches so the injured player should always see a health worker quickly.

Sprains and bruises should be treated with an ice pack or icy water to reduce the swelling. People with serious injuries like broken limbs should always be sent straight to the hospital or health centre.

Cooling down

When the game is finished and you have shaken hands with the opposition team, take time to stretch and cool down with light jogging. This is a very important part of looking after your body.

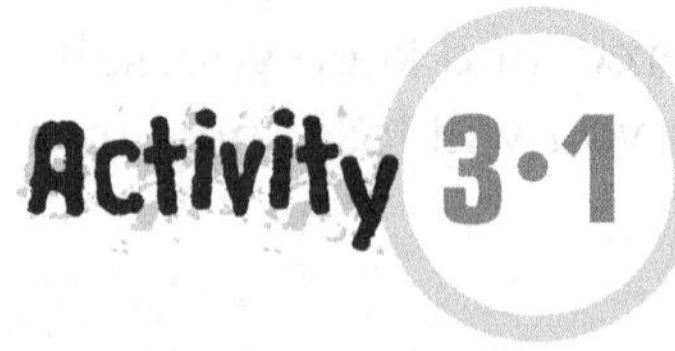

1. List the games that are played in your village. Include the made-up or traditional games as well as the formal games like soccer.
2. For each game, write down the rules that keep the players safe.
3. Which games are most unsafe? Why?
4. Finally, work with three friends to write a code of behaviour for recess play at school.

Keeping safe at play

Playing in the garden and the bush is great fun, but there are some dangerous situations that could lead to serious injuries. The best strategy is to avoid accidents when playing by careful decision-making and self-control.

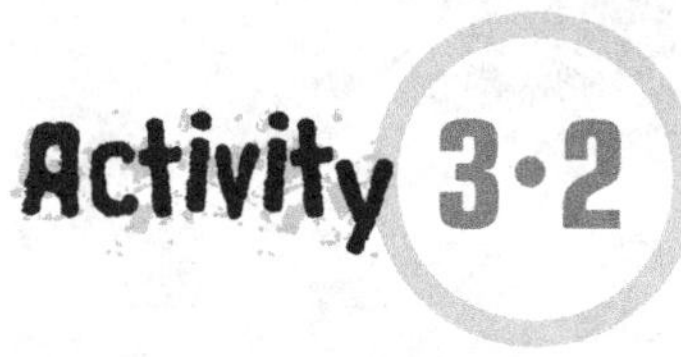

1 Select an unsafe situation that might occur when you are playing and make a poster for younger students to warn them of the dangers.
2 Make sure your poster shows the correct safe behaviour as well as the hazard. The unsafe situation should be one that is likely to happen in your own community or environment.

Dangerous animals and plants

There are many poisonous and dangerous animals and plants in PNG.

In the sea or rivers, stings and spines can be treated with hot water and vinegar. Crocodiles kill several people a year in PNG and should be treated very carefully indeed. Do not swim where they have been seen. Shark attacks are extremely rare.

In the forest or bush, local elders will be able to tell you which plants and mushrooms are poisonous.

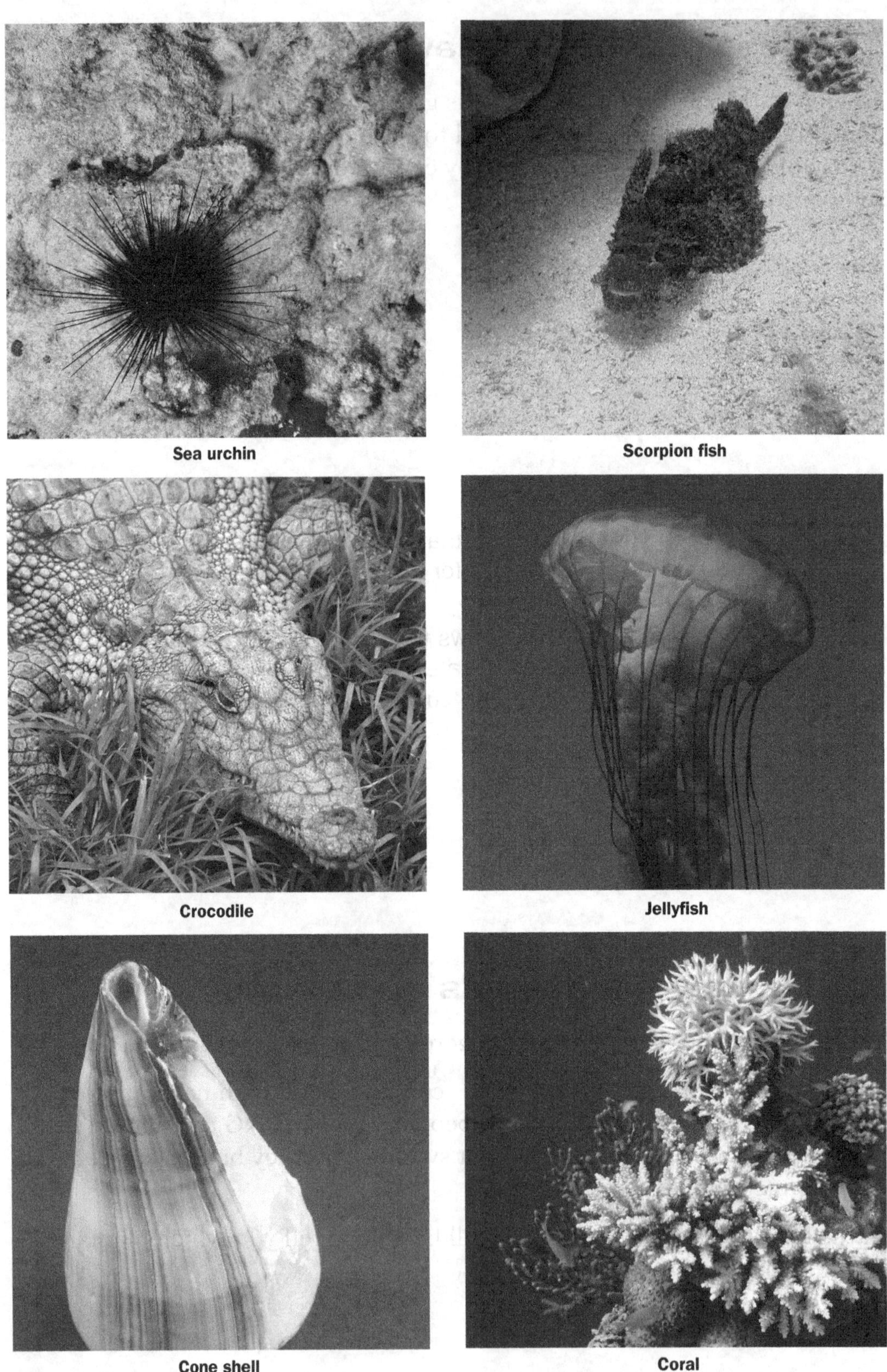
Sea urchin

Scorpion fish

Crocodile

Jellyfish

Cone shell

Coral

Snakebite

Snakes are common in PNG and are often found where children like to play. Most communities will know of people bitten by snakes. Snakes bite people because they have been frightened. Not all snakes are poisonous but some, like the Papuan taipan, are extremely dangerous.

The best way of treating snake bites is not to get bitten in the first place. Be careful around long grass, animal burrows and when looking under corrugated iron, wood piles and other materials. Snakes also like sunbathing on trails and paths, so look down where you are running or walking. If you give a snake enough warning by making noise, it will move away from you. It doesn't want to kill you. Do not chase, hunt or kill snakes. Run away if you see one.

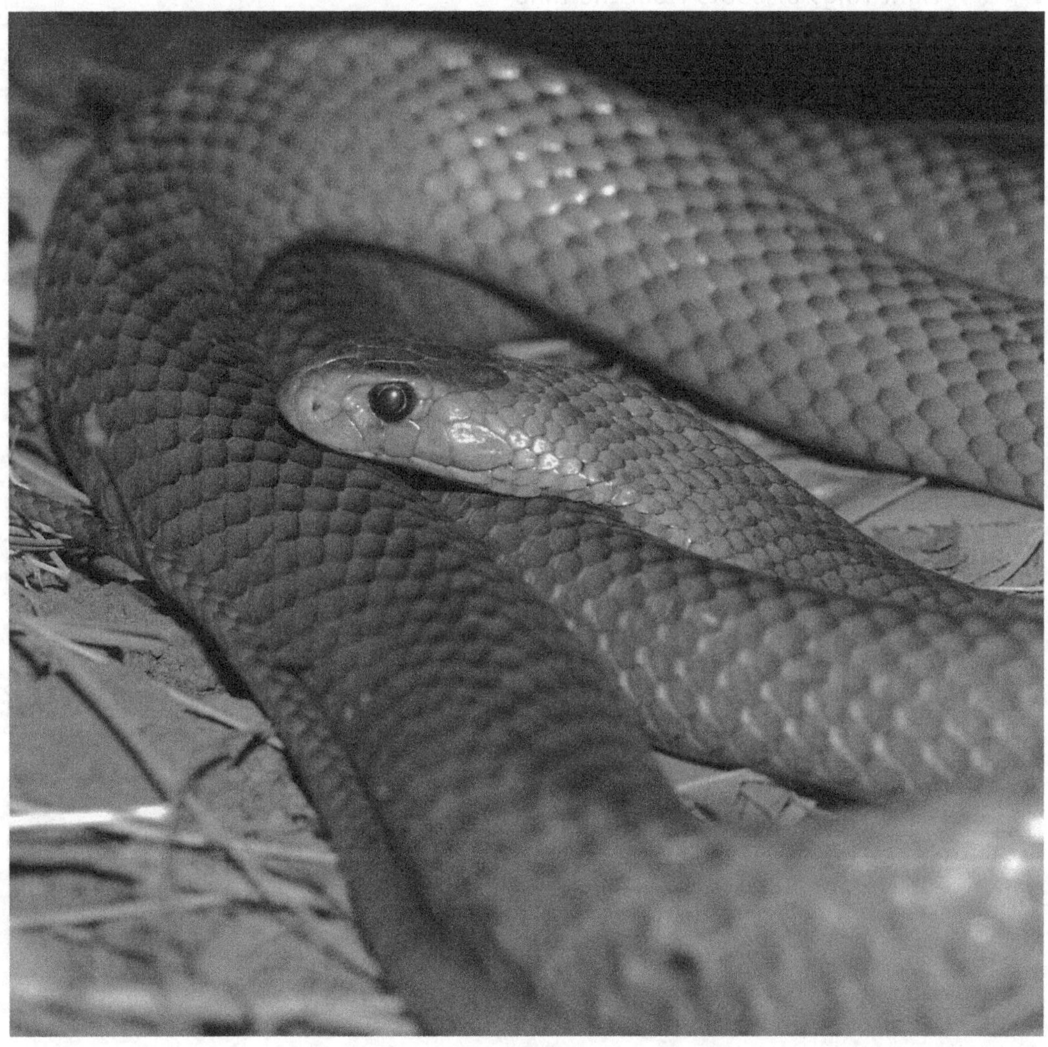

Taipan

It is important that everyone knows what to do if you or a friend are bitten by a snake.

Do:

- ☑ stay calm and stay away from the snake
- ☑ try and remember what the snake looks like but treat all snake bites as dangerous
- ☑ keep the patient calm and still, lay them down and remove any tight rings or boots from the limb
- ☑ wrap a wide pressure bandage around the limb as quickly as possible (a sheet, a *lap lap* or towel) and make sure this does not cut off the blood flow
- ☑ put the limb in a splint (use a stick, broom handle, long bush knife) so it cannot move and the poison is not pumped around the body
- ☑ get help and get the patient to an aid post as quickly as possible
- ☑ carry the patient on a stretcher if necessary
- ☑ remember that anti-venom for poisonous snakes should be available in the nearest hospital (this is a special medicine for the effects of snakebite).

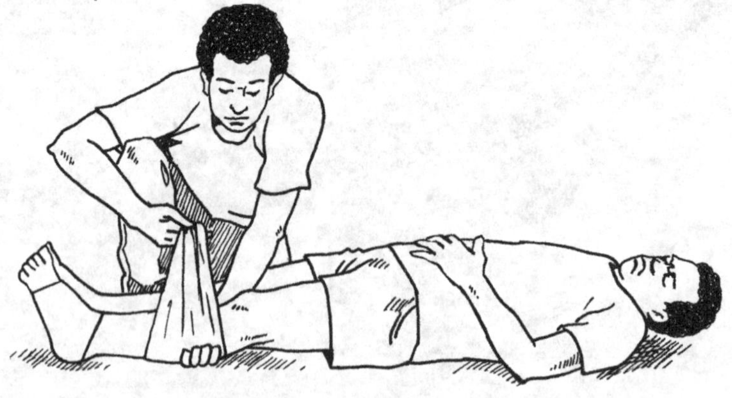

Do not:

- ☒ chase the snake or try and catch or kill the snake – it might bite someone else
- ☒ try and suck the venom out
- ☒ wash or put ice on the wound
- ☒ allow the patient to move
- ☒ cut or bleed the wound or lift the limb up
- ☒ use a tourniquet (a tight rope or rubber band) to tie up the limb
- ☒ use traditional herbs, potions or spells.

Activity 3·3

1. With two friends, role-play what to do if someone gets bitten by a snake when you are playing.
2. Make sure you include all the steps and act calmly and quickly. Remember that speed is important. Ask another friend to assess your actions.

Chapter 4 Safety at home

The home and the garden are usually safe places, but there are some potential hazards that could cause harm.

 Fire

Fire is a serious hazard in homes. Most houses in PNG are made of wood and bush materials. Many people use kerosene lamps and candles and cook on open fires. Everyone must be careful with lit lamps and fires. Never put the wrong fuel in kerosene lamps or stoves, and never leave a naked flame in the house when people are asleep. Don't let anyone smoke in the house. If you have an open fire in the house, it is a good idea to keep a covered bucket of water nearby.

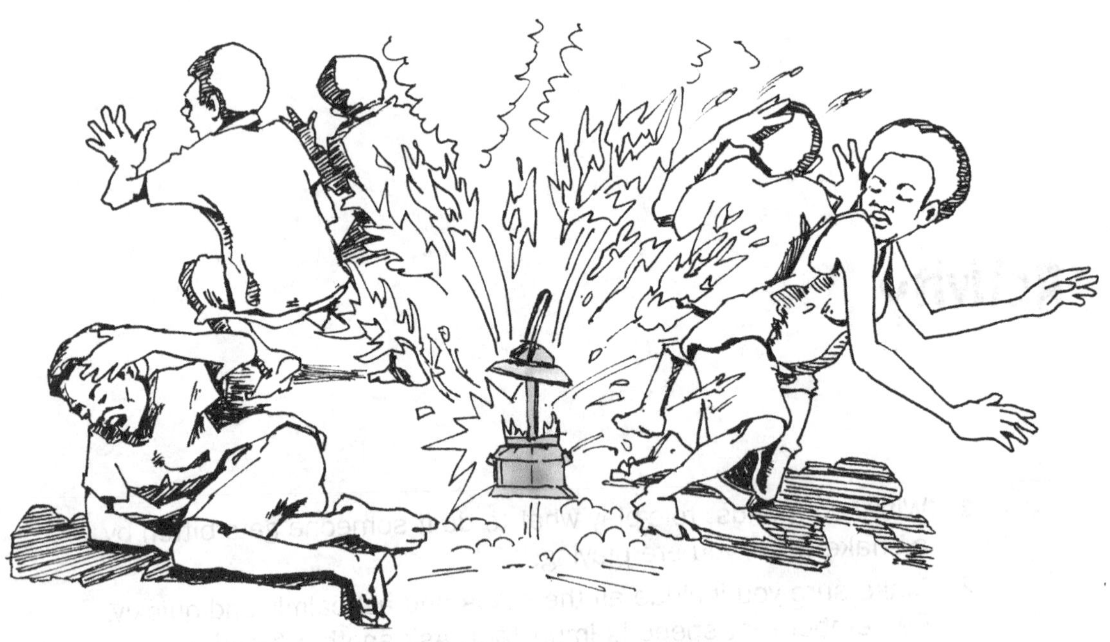

Be careful with polyester clothes and foam mattresses. They burn and melt quickly and the smoke they produce is very poisonous. It is also dangerous to you and the environment to burn plastics on open fires.

What to do in a fire

1. Warn others. Shout "fire!" to wake everybody up and get help.
2. Get yourself and others out of the house as quickly as possible.
3. Stay low to breath clean air.
4. Don't try to save possessions.
5. If you have a chance of putting the fire out, act quickly.
6. Once you and your family are out, stay out. Don't go back inside the burning house.
7. If a person's clothes have caught fire, stop them moving, drop them to the ground, wrap them in a woollen coat or blanket if possible, and roll them over to put the flames out.

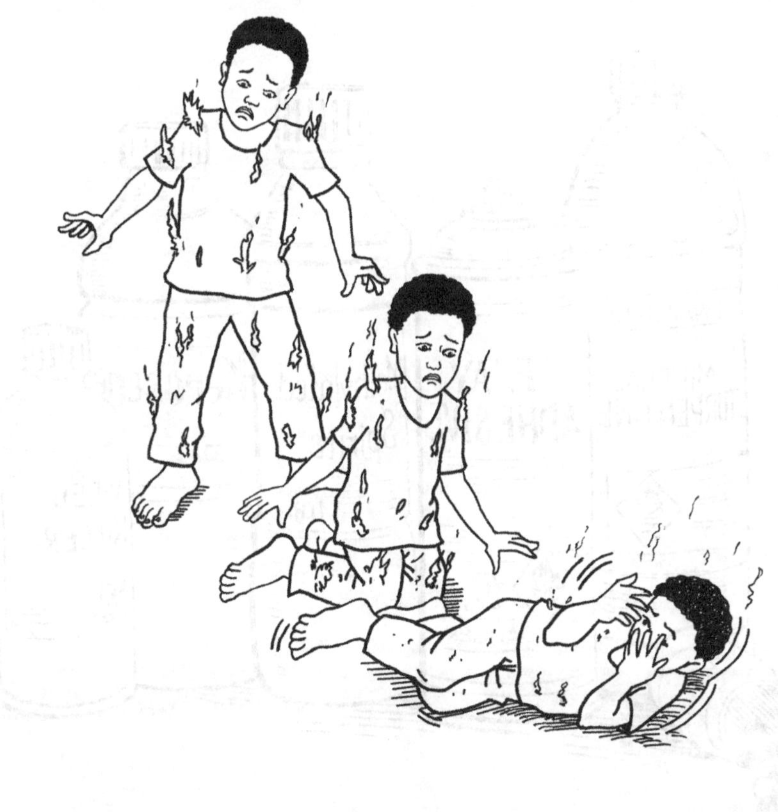

Knives and axes

Many injuries are caused by accidents with knives and axes. Always be careful when cutting grass or chopping wood. Make sure you have plenty of space around you. Keep the blade sharp and clean and keep the handle dry. If you get cut, put pressure on the wound to slow the bleeding and seek medical attention. Cuts can lead to nasty infections. Always remember to keep sharp blades away from babies and little children.

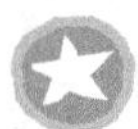

Pesticides and poisons

Many people in PNG are farmers. They keep pesticides and poisons in the house and garden to use on their crops or to get rid of pests like rats and cockroaches. Many of these are toxic chemicals and should be treated very carefully indeed.

Children will sometimes play with bleach and other cleaning fluids. This is dangerous. If a child splashes bleach into an eye or on the skin, wash the affected area with lots of clean water. If they drink bleach, you should rush them to a health centre.

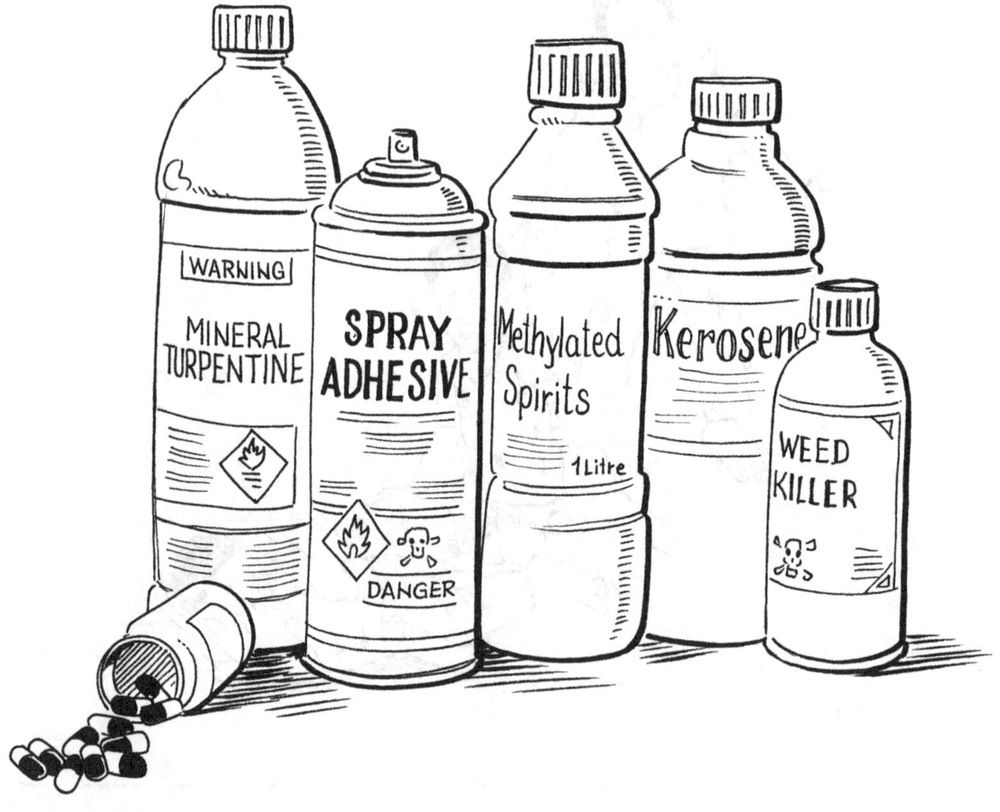

What to do with poisons

- Keep them locked away or in secure containers on a shelf away from children.
- Be careful when you throw away old poison or pesticide containers so children do not play with them.
- Farmers should use face masks when spraying. Don't breathe in the chemicals and keep children away from the sprayer.
- Only use chemicals according to the instructions and mix them up carefully.
- If your skin is irritated or you get burnt by chemicals, wash the wound with lots of clean water and go to the health centre immediately.
- If a child eats or drinks poison or pesticide, you must take them to the health centre immediately.

Medicines

Medicines have many benefits but they can be dangerous if they are not used properly. Only buy prescription medicines from a pharmacy or from a health centre (malaria medicines, worming pills, strong painkillers, antibiotics, etc.). Never buy prescription medicines from the market or street sellers because they might be stolen, out of date or fake. Medicines are designed to treat specific illnesses. Don't take prescription medicines unless a health worker has told you to.

Electricity

Electricity is extremely dangerous. An electric shock can stop your heart beating and burn you badly.

Power lines carry very powerful electrical currents. If you touch the power lines, you will be killed. Never climb power poles or go near fallen cables. Never throw anything at power cables or transformer stations. If you see a fallen cable, tell a trusted adult or the electricity company immediately. Don't throw old shoes over the power cables because someone from the power company will have to climb up and take them down.

There might be electrical equipment like toasters, kettles or televisions in the house. Keep them away from water sources, open windows and leaking roofs. Never switch on electrical equipment if you have wet hands. Always use the correct fuse and don't use equipment if the wires are frayed or split. Never let small children stick anything into electrical sockets. Regularly check that rats have not chewed through electrical cables.

If you see someone who has been electrocuted, remember to keep yourself safe first. Do not touch them. Try and turn off the electricity at the socket. If you cannot do that, use a wooden stick (wood doesn't conduct electricity) to push them away from the source of the electricity.

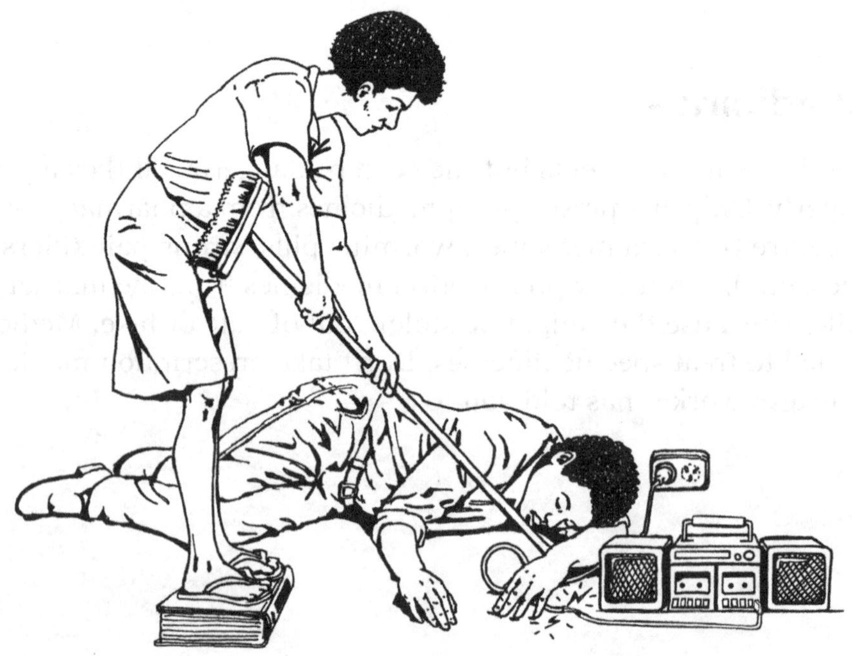

Food and drink

Dirty water and infected food cause many illnesses every year. Diarrhoea can kill small children and elderly people and makes everyone weak and sick. You and your family can easily prevent this by cooking food carefully, keeping flies off food with a net, and making sure you have clean fresh water. There should not be any cockroach or rat droppings in the kitchen area.

Malaria

The malaria parasite is transmitted to humans by mosquitoes. Malaria is a very serious disease and can kill. It is also a preventable disease.

How to prevent malaria

- Sleep under a treated bed net (mosquitoes bite at night) and put screens on your doors and windows.
- Cut long grass and fit screens on water tanks and barrels.
- If you get malaria, see a health worker for the correct medicines and always complete the course of anti-malarial drugs.
- Clean up standing water where mosquitoes breed, such as in old coconuts, cans, bottles, drains and plastic wrappers.
- Use insecticide sprays to kill mosquitoes in the house.

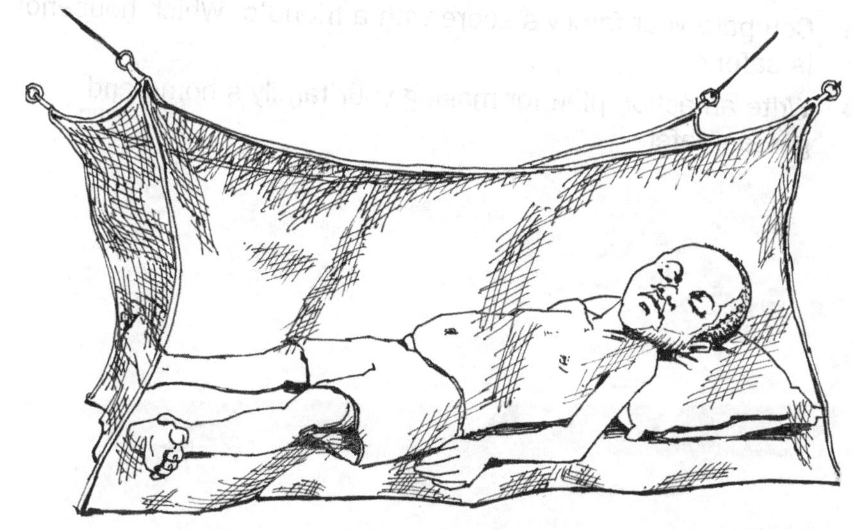

Rubbish and waste

Make sure that latrines are built a long way from community water sources like wells and rivers.

Man-made rubbish should be buried or burned in a pit so it doesn't attract pests like rats. Plastics should only be burnt outside. Litter around a house is a sign that the people who live there are not taking their health and safety seriously.

You should never throw batteries, bottles or aerosol cans into a fire because they can explode. Batteries and plastics contain toxic chemicals.

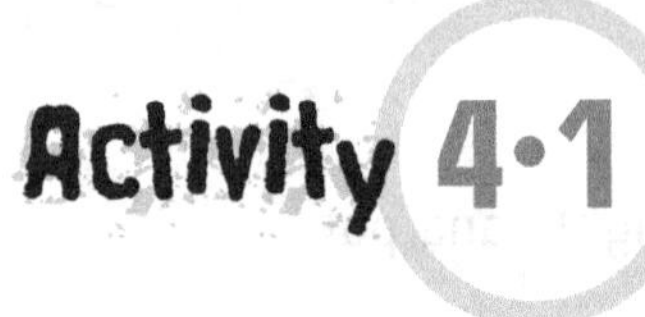

1. Survey your home and garden for the eight categories listed in this chapter.
2. Give your family a score out of five for each category.
   5 = No risk: our family is safe and protected.
   0 = Oh no! There is danger for our family
3. Compare your family's score with a friend's. Which household is safer?
4. Write an action plan for making your family's home and garden safer.

Chapter 5 Safety at school

It is really important that all children in PNG go to school, so they can learn and contribute to the development of the country. Schools should be safe, healthy and happy places to learn. Communities should support their children to go to school and they should support the teachers in their work. Every child has the right to go to school.

Everyone (teachers, students, community members) has the responsibility to make school a safe, child-friendly place.

 What makes a school unsafe?

Bullying

Bullying is when a student is made to feel unhappy or hurt by the words or actions of another student. Bullying can be physical, emotional or verbal. It is an abuse of power over someone else. Students who are bullied do not do well at school and might even stop coming to class. Anyone can be bullied.

Bullying is very harmful and it is the fault of the bully, not the victim. Bullying is a disciplinary offence in all schools and should be treated seriously by teachers and head teachers.

You should always take action to stop bullying. If you see someone being bullied, you should tell a teacher. If you are being bullied, you should ask for help. If your friend is bullying someone, make them stop. Everyone has the right to a safe school.

Activity 5•1

1 With a group of friends, list actions that are considered to be bullying.
2 Now sort the list into "most serious" and "least serious".
3 Put a tick next to every action you have witnessed in your school or class.

"I just keep the class in control. If someone is not working, I give them a slap on the ear." **Elisabeth**

"I won't play with that girl because her mother is a bad woman. When that girl comes over near me, I pinch my nose and my friends laugh." **Sali**

"When Charles is being teased, I just play along with the others. I feel bad for him but he is from another village." **Thomas**

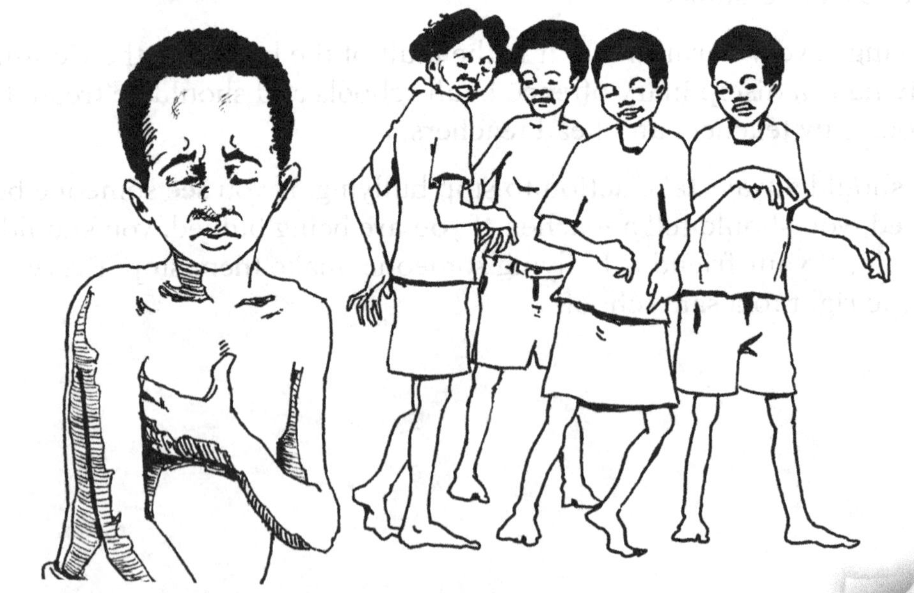

Activity 5·2

1 Read the quotes on the previous page. Are these actions bullying?

2 What should we do to reduce bullying? List at least three practical strategies for each situation.

- What I can do:
- What the teacher can do:
- What the head teacher can do:

Activity 5·3

With a partner, read the following case studies. Decide on the best course of action and what the consequences could be.

- You have started at a new primary school. In the class, there is one girl who is cruel to another. The other students don't seem to be doing anything. What do you do?
- A classmate who is stronger than you keeps punching you on the arm whenever the teacher is not looking. It hurts. What do you do?
- A peer in the dormitory keeps playing loud music late into the night. When you ask them to stop, they start calling you insulting names and telling stories about you. What do you do?

- Your teacher keeps calling you a troublemaker and punishing you for things the other students do. What do you do?
- A boy in your class makes all the girls do the cleaning of the classroom. What do you do?
- A friend comes to you crying and says that an older student pinched her and threatened her. She is lonely and frightened. What do you do?
- In class, one of the boys makes a funny comment about a girl's breasts. She is obviously upset and doesn't come to school the next day. What do you do?
- Your peer group doesn't want you to play soccer with them anymore. They say you are not very good. What do you do?
- When your group is working on their garden, a classmate accuses you of stealing their bush knife and calls you a thief. You didn't take the knife. What do you do?
- A teacher slaps your hand with a ruler for a mistake you made. This teacher often hits students. What do you do?

Poor teachers

Teachers have a responsibility to care for their students and teach them the skills, knowledge and attitudes they need to develop. Most teachers are dedicated and kind. However, some teachers do not behave well.

- They might be absent from the class a lot or turn up late for lessons.
- They don't plan or teach good lessons.
- They have favourite students.
- They pick on students unfairly.
- They are cruel or sarcastic.
- They hit or cane students.
- They might sexually harass, touch or even rape students.

Teachers should never set cruel or harmful punishments and teachers are never allowed to hit or cane students. This is against the law. Your family and the head teacher should be told immediately.

A teacher should never touch your body in a sexual way or try to have a sexual relationship with you. If a teacher has sex with a student, it is rape and a criminal offence. Your family, the police and the head teacher should be told immediately.

Peer pressure

Peer pressure can be positive or negative. Dangerous peer pressure is when your friends persuade you to take risks such as drinking home-brew or smoking. Some activities could lead to ill health or diseases such as HIV/AIDS, or get you into trouble at school or with the community.

It is important that young people know how to resist peer pressure by using the life skills of decision-making and assertiveness. Saying "no" to risky behaviour is difficult if all your friends are doing it. You need to practise these skills and be prepared for unsafe situations. You should also choose your friends carefully. A good friend will not put pressure on you.

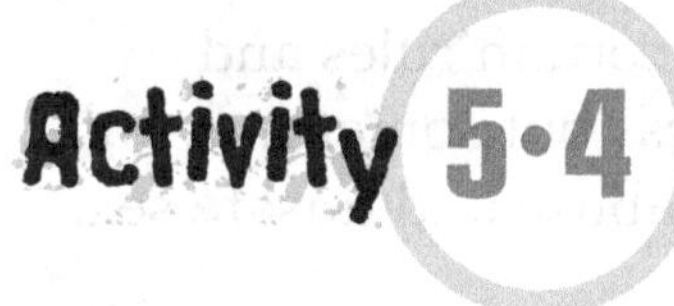

Read the questions and statements on the following page. Role-play an assertive answer, what your friend might say to persuade you and what you would say to finish the conversation. Don't forget to say the word "no", and give a strong reason for your decision!

For example:

Your friend says: "Hey, we're taking the morning off school to spin around town."

You would say: "No, my parents saved up to send me to school. I don't want to let them down."

Your friend says: "It's only one morning. All of us are going. Your parents would never find out."

You would finish the conversation by saying: "No. You go if you want, but I don't want to get into trouble and I don't want to miss my lessons."

- Your friend says: "You can't get pregnant the first time you have sex, so don't worry."
- Your friend says: "Here, have a smoke."
- Your friend says: "Look at her. She's ugly."
- Your friend says: "What's the answer to question ten?"
- Your friend says: "We're spinning down to the club to look for women. You want to come?"

Generation names and school cults

Generation names are passed down from older students to younger students. They are usually secret and are often linked to risky behaviour, such as fighting. Students are pressured by their peers to take part.

Cults are peer groups that meet in secret and have certain rules and initiation ceremonies. Sometimes these are harmless but sometimes cults can include bad behaviour, drinking alcohol, drug abuse and unsafe sex. Generation names can be part of these cults.

Many secondary schools have had problems with generation names and cults. Younger students are vulnerable when they first arrive at a secondary school. However, many students refuse to take part in generation names. Schools will discipline or expel any students taking part.

Activity 5·5

1. If you were going to secondary school, how would you resist the pressure to have a generation name?
2. List strategies for resisting the pressure and at least five alternatives to cult activity.
3. Discuss with a friend why students at secondary schools might want to be involved in cult or generation name activity. List as many reasons as you can.

Activity 5·6

Imagine you had to build the perfect child-friendly school.

1. What would the school rules be?
2. What rewards would there be for positive behaviour?
3. What would the punishments be for poor behaviour?
4. How would you make the school environment safe and healthy?
5. What kind of teachers would you recruit for your school?

Chapter 6 Travelling safely

Travelling away from home and your community is usually interesting and exciting. You might be going to stay with relatives, travelling to a new school or even moving to a new village. You might have to travel for work. However, travel in PNG is difficult because the environment is very rugged. There are huge mountains, tropical seas, fast-flowing rivers and poor roads.

 Road safety

Around the world, one of the biggest killers of children is road traffic accidents. Cars, trucks, buses and PMVs (public motor vehicles) often travel too fast, and cannot stop in time if a child is walking out into the road. At night, drivers get tired and cannot see people walking along. Some communities build speed bumps to slow down vehicles, but we must all be aware of cars and trucks when we walk along roads.

"I always walk along facing the traffic so I can see the cars coming and am ready to get out of the way." **Susi**

"I always wear a bright-coloured shirt when I am walking back home so drivers can see me when the sun is going down." **Aaron**

"I always tell my children to look right and left twice before stepping out to cross the road. I never let them cross the road on their own." **Susan**

"I bought my son and daughter a bicycle. I also taught them to ride it carefully and close to the edge of the road and look over their shoulder before pedalling out." **Henry**

Mother and child killed by racing PMV

Police are hunting for the driver of a PMV which lost control and crashed into another vehicle. The accident killed a mother and her five year old boy.

Injured passengers and pedestrians were rushed to hospital. The driver of the PMV fled into the bush. Angry relatives pulled the bus crew out of the PMV and beat them before police arrived.

Police say they expect to arrest the driver soon.

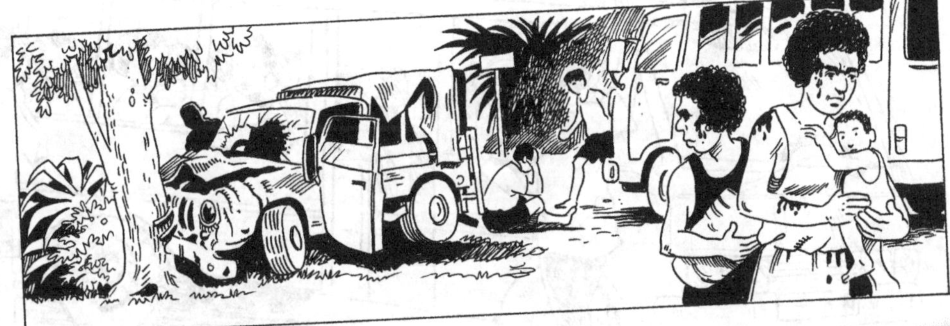

Activity 5·6

1. Read the story above.
2. What do you think happened? What other stories like it have you heard recently?
3. Do you know of any road traffic accidents that have affected your family or community?
4. Now rewrite the newspaper story with a happy ending.

Safe travel by car or PMV depends on your good decision-making. You can prepare well by choosing a good, sober driver and a trustworthy PMV and not travelling at night or on a Friday. If you are making a long journey, make sure you have water, a hat, toilet paper and something to eat in case the bus breaks down. Make sure someone knows you are coming and what time to expect you. If you have a mobile phone, make sure you have credit, and keep in contact with your relatives.

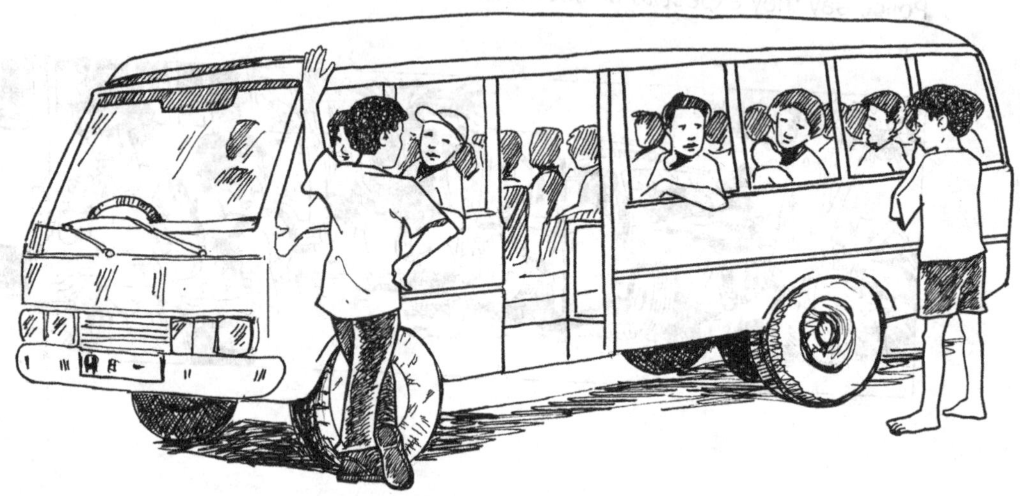

Never accept a lift from someone you do not know or trust. Never get into a vehicle that is full of people who have been drinking. If you feel uncomfortable or scared, don't get in or get out again quickly. Travel with a friend or family member if you can. Ask yourself these questions:

- Is the driver drunk or tired?
- Do I know and trust the people in the PMV?
- Are there women in the PMV?
- Can I wear a seatbelt?
- Is the PMV in good condition?
- Is this a good time to travel along a safe road?
- Is there a risk from *raskols*?
- Is it going to rain or am I going to get hot in the sun?

Travelling safely by dinghy

Every year, there are stories of boats going missing in the coastal seas around PNG. Sometimes the people are found and rescued. Sometimes they are never seen again.

Travelling by dinghy can be wet and cold or you could be out in the sun for a long time. Always travel with a hat, spare dry clothes wrapped in a waterproof plastic bag, and plenty of water and food. If you have a mobile phone, make sure it is turned on, has credit, and is fully charged. Don't travel by dinghy unless you can swim. It is always better to travel with a friend or family member.

If the sea is rough, the operator is drunk, or if it is late in the day or storms are expected, do not risk travelling by dinghy. Always make sure there is someone expecting you at the destination, there are calm seas and no storm warnings, and the dinghy:

- is not overloaded
- has a sober and experienced operator and crew
- has a mix of men and women
- has a well-maintained engine with spare spark plugs and tools
- has plenty of fuel
- has a plastic tarpaulin to cover cargo
- is not travelling late in the afternoon or at night
- has life jackets, an emergency radio beacon and supplies
- is travelling in a boat convoy if possible.

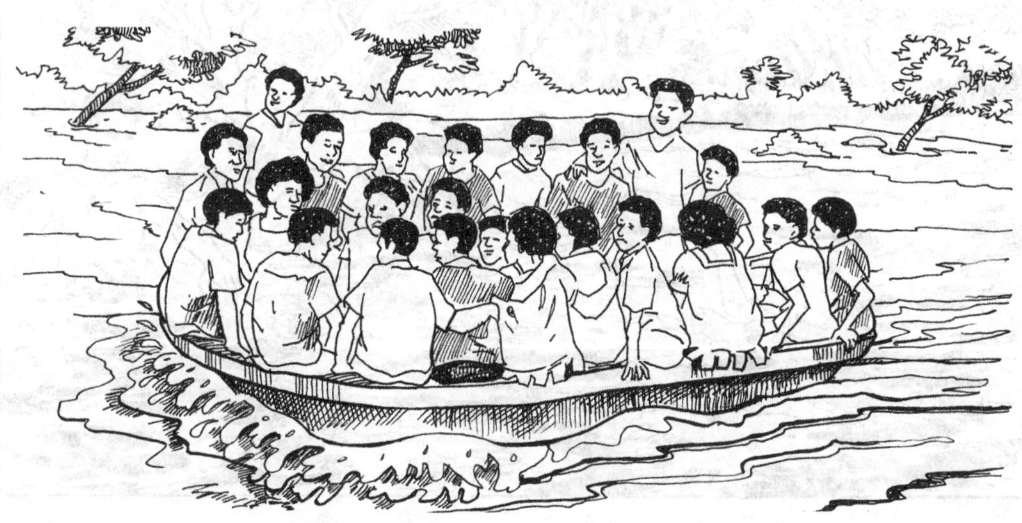

Activity 6·2

1 Write a short case study about a young person on a long dinghy or PMV journey that goes wrong.
2 Write two endings – one happy and one sad.
3 What lessons can a young person learn from your story? Make a list.

Crossing rivers safely

In tropical countries, a sudden thunderstorm in the mountains can quickly flood a river downstream. This can make rivers very dangerous to cross. Most rivers in PNG do not have bridges and the strong currents can sweep people away and drown them.

You need to be aware of the state of the river. If it is rising quickly and the water is becoming muddy and waves are appearing, it could be beginning to flood. It is safer to wait until the flood has passed than risk your life by trying to cross it.

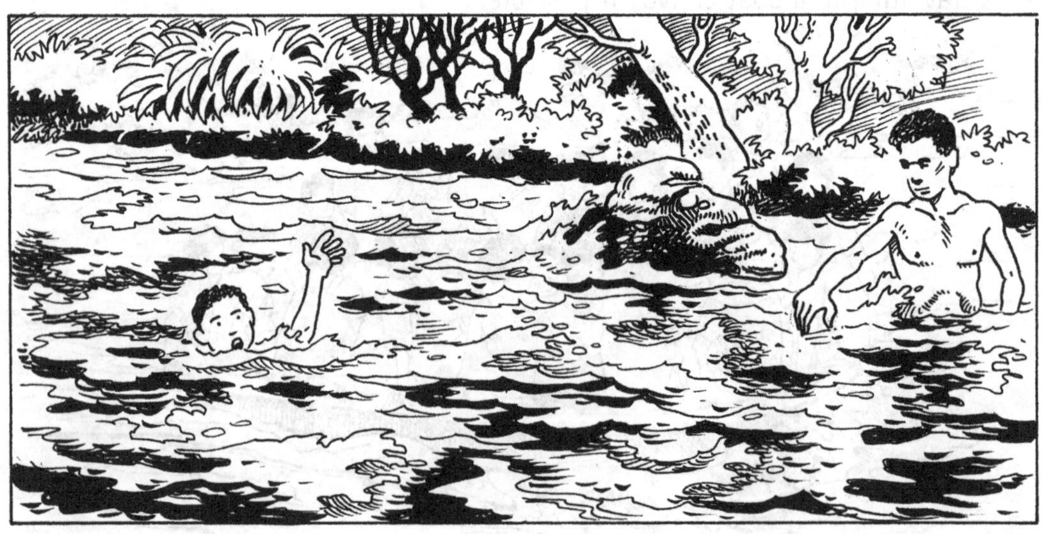

Florence's story

My primary school was a long walk from my village. I used to walk my little brother to school every day and we used to cross a wide river just before the school. All the other children from my village used to wade across the river before and after school. There was no bridge.

One day, we stayed behind after school to help plant our class garden. By the time we got to the river, it was high and fast flowing. I lifted my brother up on my shoulders and started to cross. The water was very cold and strong. The boulders in the river were tumbling along and kept knocking me over. I was very scared and my brother was crying. Once or twice I fell and the water came up to my chest.

Finally we got to the other side and lay there exhausted. My ankles and feet were bleeding badly.

Later we heard our neighbours' daughter was drowned. She had tried to cross just half an hour after us. There had been a huge storm up in the mountains that we did not see.

Activity 6·3

1 What would you have done if you were Florence? Why?
2 What caused the unsafe situation?
3 How do you think Florence felt when she heard the news about her neighbour's daughter?

The most important thing you can do to keep safe around water is to learn to swim. This skill could save your life. Ask an older brother or sister or your parents to teach you how to swim.

If you have to cross a flooded strong river, there are some strategies you can use to stop yourself being swept away.

1 Keep your shoes on if you have them to protect your feet.
2 Work as a team.
3 Use a stick to support yourself.
4 Walk downstream and find a wider place to cross.
5 If you get swept off your feet, keep your feet pointing down the river and try and paddle towards the bank.
6 Grab any floating material you can.

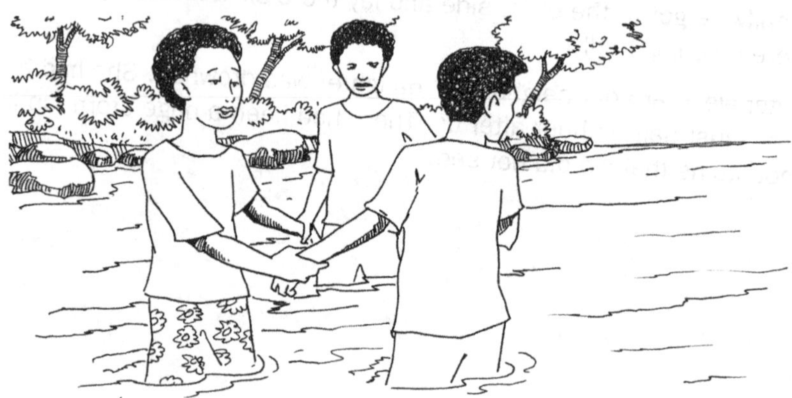

Activity 6·4

1 Work with a group of friends to write the top ten rules for safe travelling.
2 Which ones are most important? Why?
3 Which ones will you follow?
4 Which ones would you explain to younger siblings?

Chapter 7 Natural disasters

PNG is a country on the "ring of fire." There is a crack in the crust of the Earth that runs very close to our country. This means PNG has many active volcanoes and many earthquakes. Earthquakes can cause tsunamis, which are large waves that can sweep over coastal villages.

PNG also experiences tropical storms and cyclones. It has regular dry and wet seasons and there are often very strong winds. All these factors mean that everyone needs to be prepared for natural disasters and emergencies.

You and your family should talk about a disaster plan, and decide what you would you do and where you would go in an emergency. Your family should have an emergency kit including a first aid kit, a torch, spare clothes, mosquito net and emergency rations.

Activity 7·1

Make a list of the natural disasters that have affected PNG in recent years.

1 Research them by talking to adults and older people in your community.
2 Sort these natural disasters in order of the damage caused. Which ones were the most serious?
3 Discuss with a friend which natural disasters are most likely to affect your community and put your safety at risk.

Tropical storms and flooding

Tropical storms regularly batter countries in the Pacific region. There are strong winds and torrential rain. This can damage buildings, destroy food gardens and cause sudden flooding. For example, tropical cyclone Guba destroyed much of Oro Province in PNG in 2007, and washed out almost every bridge.

What to do in a tropical storm

- Keep an emergency stock of canned food, rice and several full water containers.
- Don't travel by boat or canoe when the storm is coming, and take extra care around flooded rivers.
- Make sure your house and roof are secure and tie down any loose materials.
- If necessary, move to higher ground or a more sturdy building like the church or school.
- Check on your neighbours and tell people the storm is coming.
- Stay inside when the storm is raging and only go outside in an emergency. There will be lots of debris flying around.
- Do not shelter under trees or next to electricity lines, especially if there is lightning nearby. If you are exposed out on the mountainside, lie down flat.

Bushfires

Bushfires can be man-made or natural. During the dry season, people burn long grass to clear gardens or to hunt animals. However, in strong winds bushfires can get out of control and burning ash can travel a long distance.

What to do in a bushfire

- Keep a fire break of short grass around your house and keep water nearby if the fire comes closer.
- If the fire is close to your house, wet the house with water.
- Do not light fires without a good reason and never light a bushfire on a windy day.
- Warn people if you see a fire.
- Watch out for terrified animals running away from the fire, as many people get bitten by snakes during bushfires.
- Bushfires can move very quickly in strong wind so keep your distance.

 Landslides

Landslides can happen after heavy rain, especially on steep slopes that have been cleared for gardens. The famous Highlands Highway in PNG is frequently cut by landslides caused by blocked drains and unstable mountainsides. Earthquakes can also cause landslides.

Large landslides can sweep away whole villages and bury people beneath mud and debris. The best way of reducing risk from landslides is to build your house in a safe place away from steep slopes and not to cut the trees from the hillside. Care should be taken when making gardens or logging, so the hill does not become eroded and the soil does not wash away. Once the vegetation is removed, steep hillsides will be vulnerable to landslides.

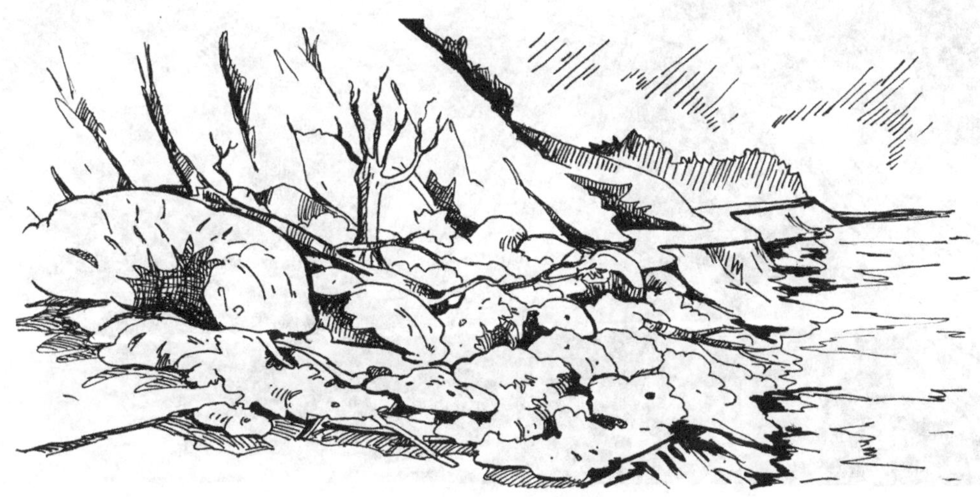

Earthquakes

An earthquake happens when the giant plates that make up the Earth's crust jolt against each other. Very powerful forces are released which suddenly make the ground move and heave. This shaking movement can destroy buildings, cause tsunamis, trigger landslides and seriously damage towns and roads.

Most earthquakes are small and do little or no damage, but once in a while there will be an extremely powerful earthquake. PNG experiences some very strong and frequent earthquakes. There is no way to predict when an earthquake will happen.

What to do in an earthquake

- If you are inside a building during an earthquake, run outside immediately if you can and stay away from the building until the tremors stop.
- If you can't get outside, hide under a strong table or door frame.
- Keep away from windows that might shatter.
- If you live on the coast, move to higher ground and help others to do the same in case a tsunami occurs.
- Get away from steep hillsides and tall buildings.
- Watch out for water tanks – they can burst open because of the shaking.
- There may be aftershocks so be prepared with emergency rations and water.

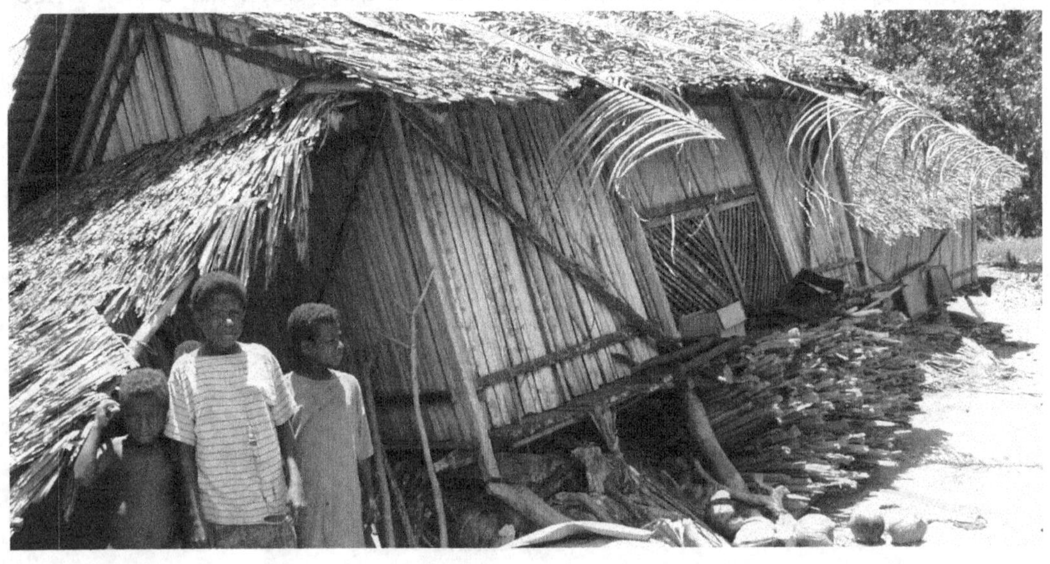

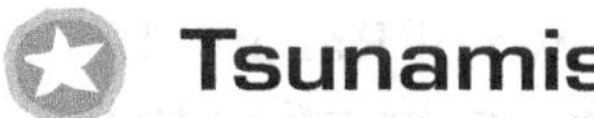

Tsunamis

A tsunami is sometimes called a "tidal wave". It is a series of large waves produced by a powerful earthquake under the ocean. Out at sea, these waves look very small, but when they reach the shore they become huge and powerful and can destroy coastal villages.

In 1998, a tsunami in Aitape killed several thousand people and devastated many communities.

The signs of a tsunami are easy to spot:

- there is a powerful earthquake
- the sea often runs away from the beach
- there is a sudden roaring and a lot of surf on the reef.

What to do in a tsunami

- If you see signs of a tsunami, warn other people and run away as fast as you can to higher ground at least 500 to 1000 metres from the beach.
- Don't stop to collect possessions and don't stop to look.
- If you cannot run to higher ground, climb strong buildings or trees.
- Many people are killed by the debris washing back out to sea after the tsunami, so try and get above the water level.
- Listen for the all-clear on the radio and go and help others.
- There may be several more waves, so be careful.

Volcanoes

PNG has some of the most active and violent volcanoes in the world. People like to live near them because the soil is very fertile. However, volcanoes can erupt without warning.

Volcanoes produce molten rock called lava, as well as choking ash and burning rock. The ash can cause huge mudslides. Some of PNG's volcanoes also erupt in the form of pyroclastic flows. These are fast-moving clouds of burning gas and ash that flow quickly down the slopes of the volcano. These flows are extremely dangerous.

In 1994, a powerful volcanic eruption destroyed the town of Rabaul. In 2004 and 2005, the people of Manam Island had to flee an eruption that devastated their island. In the last 100 years, there have been many deaths and much damage caused by volcanoes.

If you live near an active volcano, you must always be prepared for an eruption even if the volcano looks dormant. Never ever climb into the crater of a volcano because there may be invisible poisonous gases there.

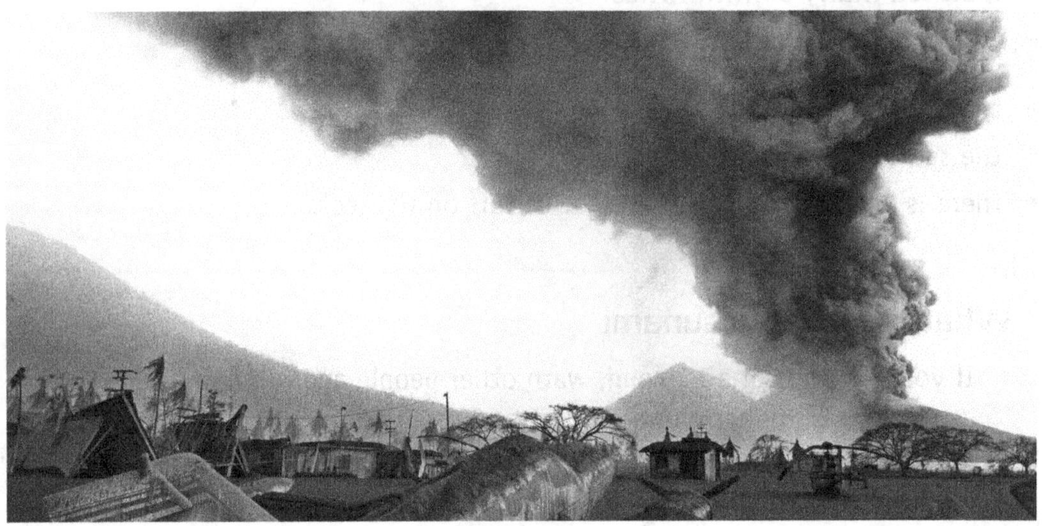

What to do if a volcano erupts

- Prepare and practise an evacuation plan.
- Keep emergency supplies, a torch and water in the house and listen to advice from the Disaster Committee.
- Use a mask to protect your lungs from the ash and cover up when you leave the house.
- You will need a torch with spare batteries because of the ash fall.
- Sweep any ash off your roof immediately and shelter inside your house unless there is an evacuation.
- Stay away from the eruption and rivers or channels that could become mud flows or landslides.
- Never damage the volcano monitoring equipment or steal the solar panels that power the sensors. Protect the equipment and the scientists might be able to warn your community before an eruption begins.

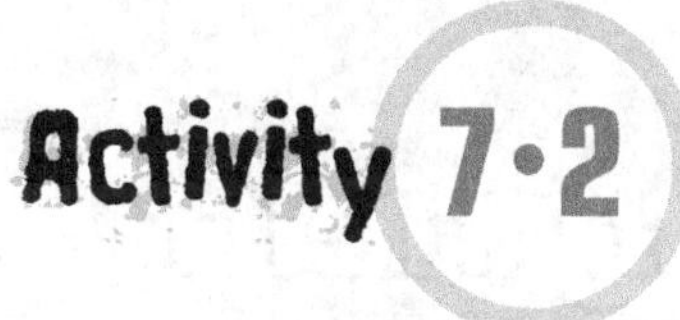

1. Select the one natural disaster that is most likely to affect you and your family in the place where you live.
2. Prepare an action plan and list what you will need to have in your emergency kit.

NATURAL DISASTER PLAN

In case of a natural disaster, our family will:

1 ______________________________

2 ______________________________

3 ______________________________

4 ______________________________

5 ______________________________

In our emergency kit, we will keep:

____

____

In an evacuation, we will remember to take:

____

____

Chapter 8 Getting help

If you have to tell someone about an emergency or an accident, you need to keep calm and give the correct information. It is hard to be calm when you are running to the health centre or someone is badly hurt. But it is important you warn adults and give them the correct information.

Always remember to give the most important information first:

- Who is hurt?
- What is the injury or danger?
- Where is the injured person or the danger?
- When did it happen?
- What help do you need?

"Help! Jacob was swept away in the river by the mango tree ten minutes ago and we can't see him. Please come and help us!" **Simon**

"Please help me! Edoa was playing rugby touch at the school field and smashed her head. It is bleeding badly and she is unconscious. We need a nurse. Please come quickly." **Cathy**

"Fire! Fire! Our house is on fire! Please come and help! I cannot find my baby brother, Daniel." **John**

"Help me! Protect me! A man tried to grab me on the path down by the creek. I ran away. Keep me safe!" **Sarah**

"Help! Daisy has been bitten by a snake in the cemetery just a few minutes ago. She is lying still and we have wrapped her leg with a *lap lap*. Please come quickly and help us carry her. It is an emergency." **Kali**

If you have to use a telephone to pass on a message, stay calm and talk loudly and slowly. Always give your name and your phone number first in case you run out of credit. Answer the questions of the doctor or the police officer. Give the important information: who, what, where, when and how. Make sure the person on the other end of the phone knows that you need help.

"Help! I am Brenda Kali calling from Takuaba village. My number is 72512345. We need the police quickly. My uncle is attacking my mother and hitting her. He is drunk. We need help. Please come quickly!"

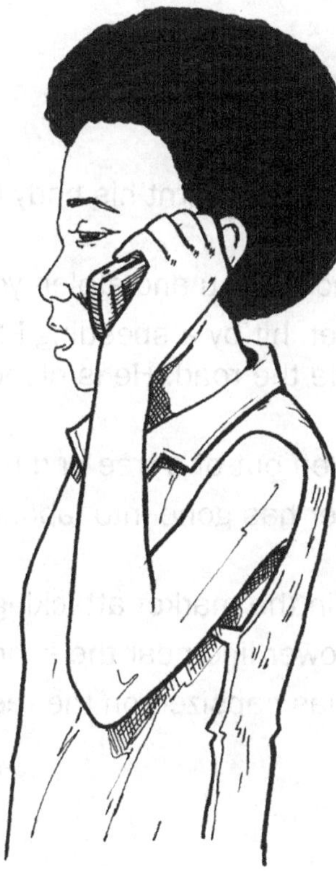

Emergency contact numbers

Emergency numbers can be found in the front of the telephone book. For an ambulance you should phone **111**.

Activity 8·1

Read the following emergency situations. Working with a friend, practise what you would say to a trusted adult if these situations happened. Role-play the situation two or three times to make sure you include all the correct details. Your friend can assess how calm you are, how urgent your information is and whether you ask clearly for the help that you need.

1 Your younger brother has burnt his body badly by falling into the fire.
2 Someone has attacked you and stolen your bilum.
3 Your friend has been hit by a speeding PMV and is unconscious beside the road. He is bleeding badly. Call an ambulance.
4 Your sister has fallen out of a tree and badly broken her arm.
5 Your pregnant sister has gone into labour in the house and is screaming in pain.
6 A drunken man is in the market attacking the mothers.
7 There is a fallen power line near the school. Call the police.
8 The boat to town has capsized on the reef and all the people are in the sea.

Activity 8·2

Use the following table to record the correct contact names, location and phone numbers (if possible) for people you might contact in an emergency.

Emergency contact	Name	Location	Phone number
Local police officer			
Nearest police station			
Local health worker			
Nearest health centre (aid post or hospital)			
Trusted adult			
Teacher or school-based counsellor			

Chapter 9 What have we learnt?

Safety is something everyone has to take responsibility for. Accidents and emergencies rarely happen, but you need to be prepared for action. You need to know about what to do and what not to do in an unsafe situation. Threats and danger need cool heads and quick decision-making. These are safety skills you can learn and practise.

If you are in danger:

1. Get away from the danger as quickly as you can.
2. Warn others.
3. Be prepared for unsafe situations and think about what you would do if there was an emergency.
4. Practise what to do in an emergency and know your first-aid skills.
5. Know someone trustworthy who you can go to for help.
6. Learn about dangerous and unsafe situations and how to avoid them.

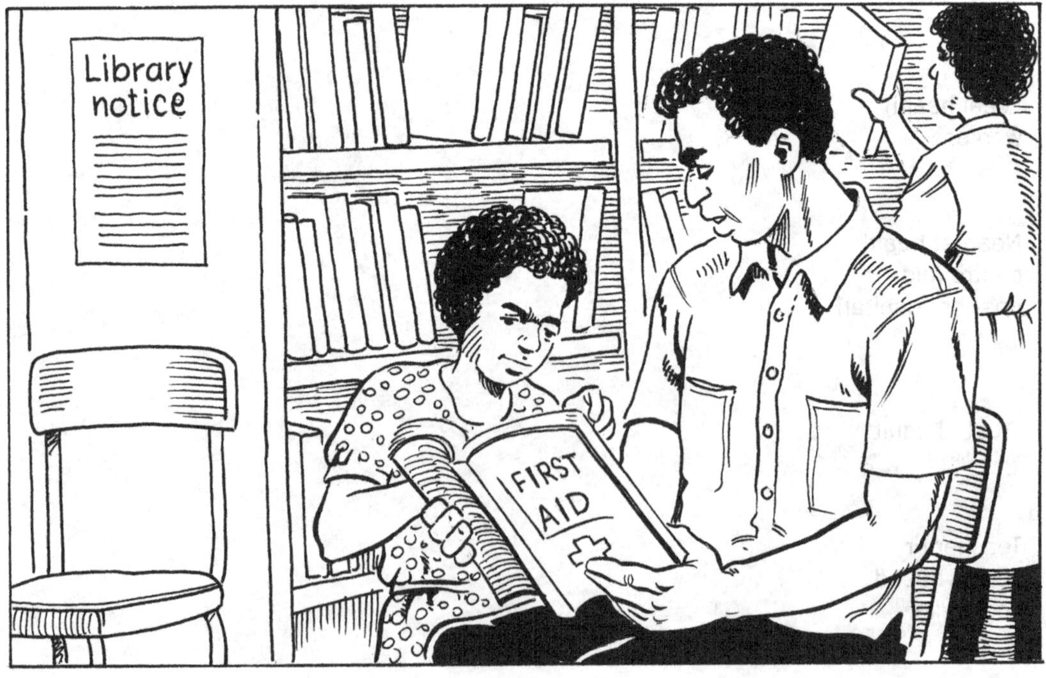

If someone else is in danger:

1 Make sure you are safe first.
2 Warn the person of the danger.
3 Help the person in danger without putting yourself at risk.
4 Practise what to do in an emergency and know your first-aid skills.
5 Get help as soon as possible.
6 Teach your younger brothers and sisters and your friends how to keep safe and avoid dangerous and unsafe situations.

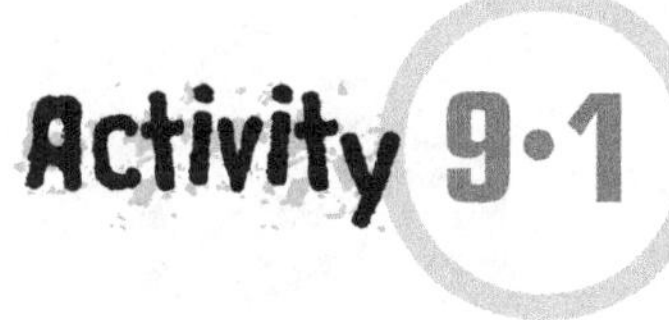

1 Ask a friend to test you on the correct and safest thing to do in different unsafe situations. For example, what is the correct plan of action for snakebite?
2 Your friend can check your responses against the information in this book.

Organisations and contacts

First Aid

St John's Ambulance
PO Box 6075, Boroko
NCD
326 2222

Red Cross Papua New Guinea
Taurama Road, Korobosea
NCD
325 8759

Kavieng 984 2116
Madang 852 2271
Rabaul 982 8580

Your local aid post or health centre can also help with teaching basic first aid skills.

Child rights

Save the Children in Papua New Guinea
PO Box 667, Goroka
732 1825

UNICEF
PO Box 472, Port Moresby
321 3000

Papua New Guinea Department of Education
Guidance Branch
PO Box 446, Waigani
325 7555

There should be trained school-based counsellors at all secondary and large town primary schools. Every Province should have welfare and guidance officers. There are also many local non-governmental organisations working with young people across the country. If you need help or advice, always speak to a trusted adult.

The United Nations Convention on the Rights of the Child

This is a simplified version of the United Nations Convention on the Rights of the Child. It has been signed by 191 countries. Papua New Guinea has signed this international agreement. There are many laws protecting the safety of children and young people in our country. You should learn your rights and your responsibilities for keeping yourself safe and healthy.

Article 1

Everyone under 18 has all these rights.

Article 2

You have the right to protection against discrimination. This means that nobody can treat you badly because of your colour, sex or religion, if you speak another language, have a disability, or are rich or poor.

Article 3

All adults should always do what is best for you.

Article 4

You have the right to have your rights made a reality by the government.

Article 5

You have the right to be given guidance by your parents and family.

Article 6

You have the right to life.

Article 7

You have the right to have a name and a nationality.

Article 8

You have the right to an identity.

Article 9

You have the right to live with your parents, unless it is bad for you.

Article 10

If you and your parents are living in separate countries, you have the right to get back together and live in the same place.

Article 11

You should not be kidnapped.

Article 12

You have the right to an opinion and for it to be listened to and taken seriously.

Article 13

You have the right to find out things and say what you think, through making art, speaking and writing, unless it breaks the rights of others.

Article 14

You have the right to think what you like and be whatever religion you want to be, with your parents' guidance.

Article 15

You have the right to be with friends and join or set up clubs, unless this breaks the rights of others.

Article 16

You have the right to a private life. For instance, you can keep a diary that other people are not allowed to see.

Article 17

You have the right to collect information from the media – radios, newspapers, television, the Internet and so on – from all around the world. You should also be protected from information that could harm you.

Article 18

You have the right to be brought up by your parents, if possible.

Article 19

You have the right to be protected from being hurt or badly treated.

Article 20

You have the right to special protection and help if you can't live with your parents.

Article 21

You have the right to have the best care for you if you are adopted or fostered or living in care.

Article 22

You have the right to special protection and help if you are a refugee. A refugee is someone who has had to leave their country because it is not safe for them to live there.

Article 23

If you are disabled, either mentally or physically, you have the right to special care and education to help you develop and lead a full life.

Article 24

You have a right to the best health possible and to medical care and to information that will help you to stay well.

Article 25
You have the right to have your living arrangements checked regularly if you have to be looked after away from home.

Article 26
You have the right to help from the government if you are poor or in need.

Article 27
You have the right to a good enough standard of living. This means you should have food, clothes and a place to live.

Article 28
You have the right to education.

Article 29
You have the right to education that tries to develop your personality and abilities as much as possible and encourages you to respect other people's rights and values and to respect the environment.

Article 30
If you come from a minority group because of your race, religion or language, you have the right to enjoy your own culture, practise your own religion, and use your own language.

Article 31
You have the right to play and relax by doing things like sports, music and drama.

Article 32
You have the right to protection from work that is bad for your health or education.

Article 33
You have the right to be protected from dangerous drugs.

Article 34
You have the right to be protected from sexual abuse.

Article 35
No one is allowed to kidnap you or sell you.

Article 36
You have the right to protection from of any other kind of exploitation.

Article 37
You have the right not to be punished in a cruel or hurtful way.

Article 38
You have a right to protection in times of war. If you are under 15, you should never have to be in an army or take part in a battle.

Article 39

You have the right to help if you have been hurt, neglected, or badly treated.

Article 40

You have the right to help in defending yourself if you are accused of breaking the law.

Article 41

You have the right to any rights in laws in your country or internationally that give you better rights than these.

Article 42

All adults and children should know about this convention. You should learn your rights and adults should learn about them too.

Adapted by Save the Children Canada from the *UN Convention on the Rights of the Child,* Office of the United Nations High Commissioner for Human Rights, © 1989 United Nations.

Glossary

anti-venom
special medicine for treating poisonous snake bites

assertiveness
saying what you want without being weak or aggressive. Assertiveness is an important life skill.

bullying
when a victim is made to feel emotional, mental or physical pain by someone else

conflict resolution
strategies for solving fights and arguments without violence

cyclone
a powerful tropical storm with strong winds, heavy rain and high tides

emergency
when a person's life or health is suddenly threatened

first aid
treating emergency injuries and sicknesses such as unconsciousness, a heart attack, broken bones, burns or bleeding

hazard
a potentially risky situation such as a flooding river or an unsafe object such as broken glass

insecticide
chemicals that kill insects such as cockroaches and other pests. Some garden insecticides are poisonous to humans.

natural disaster
a major emergency which is caused by a natural process and harms many people. For example, a tsunami or earthquake.

peer pressure
when a person's friends persuade them to do something or a person does what their friends do to be part of a group. Peer pressure can be negative or positive.

pesticide
different chemicals that kill pests on crops. Some pesticides are poisonous to humans. Insecticides and fungicides are different types of pesticide.

pyroclastic flow
a violent and dangerous cloud of burning ash and gases which travels very quickly down a volcano during an eruption

rape
when a person forces another person to have sexual intercourse (vaginal, anal or oral sex) against their will. Rape is a criminal offence.

safety
when a person is not at risk of mental, emotional or physical harm from their environment or from people

self-defence
skills used to defend yourself against a violent attack and help you escape to safety

sexual assault
when a person physically attacks another person in a sexual way. Sexual assault is a criminal offence.

sexual harassment
when a person bullies another person using sexually explicit words, jokes or sexual touching

toxic
poisonous

tsunami
a series of huge waves caused by an underwater earthquake. A tsunami is sometimes called a "tidal wave".

venom
poisons made by dangerous animals like snakes and sea urchins

Notes

Notes